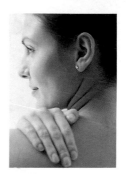

healing
hands

A concise guide to the
therapeutic power of touch

RAJE AIREY

HERMES
HOUSE

The edition published by Hermes House

© Anness Publishing Limited 2002 updated 2003..

Hermes House is an imprint of Anness Publishing Limited,
Hermes House, 88–89 Blackfriars Road, London SE1 8HA

Publisher: Joanna Lorenz
Production Controller: Joanna King

Publisher's Note:
The Reader should not regard the recommendations, ideas and techniques
expressed and described in this book as substitutes for the advice of a
qualified medical practitioner or other qualified professional.
Any use to which the recommendations, ideas and techniques
are put is at the reader's sole discretion and risk.

Printed in Hong Kong/China

3 5 7 9 10 8 6 4

contents

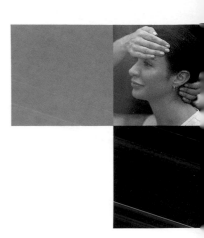

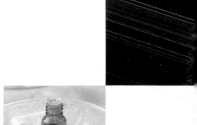

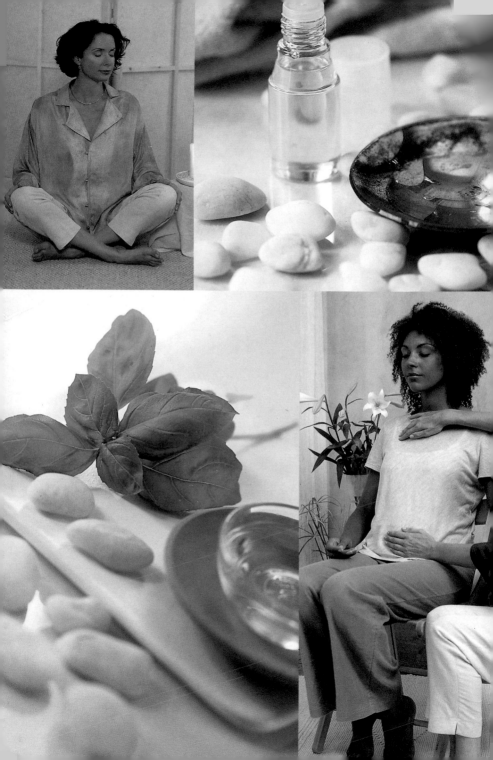

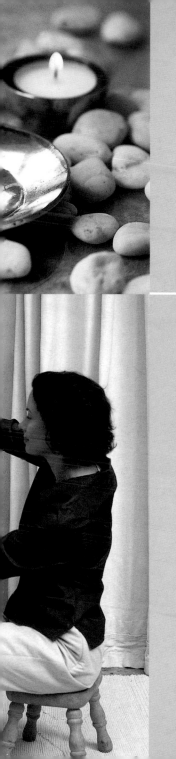

introduction

Since the earliest times, our hands have been a means of caring, comfort and giving. "Rubbing it better" is our natural response to a child's bumps and bruises and we respond to emotional pain with a hug or caress. Out of this basic instinct, healing traditions all over the world have developed their own unique systems and techniques, harnessing the power of touch to relieve pain and stimulate the body's self-healing mechanisms.

The following pages include an introduction to four well-known hands-on therapies drawn from East and West: massage, shiatsu, reflexology and reiki. With practice it is easy to include these disciplines in our daily lives, using a little healing touch to help us relax and cope with the pressures of modern living, and to treat minor ailments the drug-free way.

the power of touch

We all need to be touched in some way. Touch is a basic human instinct with the power to comfort and reassure on many levels. It can relax the body, calm the mind and encourage healing and emotional wellbeing.

A NATURAL IMPULSE

The desire to touch and be touched is one of our most instinctive needs. The sense of touch is the first to develop in the embryo, and babies thrive on close physical contact with their mothers. The caring, loving touch of another is fundamental to the development of a healthy human being. This need to be touched does not stop with the end of childhood, yet as adults many of us have become afraid to reach out and touch one another. Mistrustful of our natural loving impulse, we have lost touch with

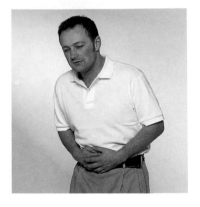

▲ IF WE FEEL PAIN OUR INSTINCT IS TO HOLD OURSELVES OR RUB THE PAIN BETTER.

ourselves and with the wisdom of the body. The beauty of practising therapeutic touch techniques is that we can begin to re-establish contact with ourselves – and others – in a way that is safe, caring and non-intrusive.

OUR SKIN

The skin is the body's largest sensory organ. By touching the skin, receptors in the dermis (the skin's second layer) react to the external stimulus and send messages through the nervous system to the

▼ YOUR BABY WILL ENJOY BEING MASSAGED AND STROKED BY YOU.

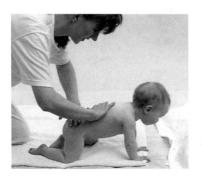

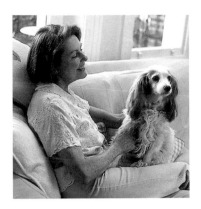

▲ PETS ENJOY A SOOTHING TOUCH JUST AS MUCH AS WE ENJOY GIVING IT.

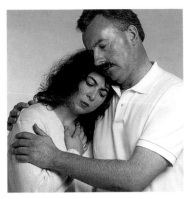

▲ IF SOMEONE CLOSE TO US IS UPSET OUR NATURAL INSTINCT IS TO GIVE THEM A HUG.

brain. A gentle stroking technique can trigger the release of endorphins, the body's natural painkillers, and induce feelings of comfort and wellbeing. More vigorous touching techniques get to work on the underlying muscular structure of the body, stretching tense and uncomfortable muscles and easing stiffness in the joints.

BENEFITS OF TOUCH

Awareness of the therapeutic value of touch is growing and many touch-therapies are widely used in conventional healthcare to treat pain, ease discomfort and to improve the functional workings of the body. Given the pressures of modern-day living and the increased incidence of stress-related illness, touch therapies also have an important part to play in everyday life. Aching backs and shoulders after a tiring day at work hunched over a computer or stood on your feet, strained leg muscles after excessive exercise, or circulatory problems from a sedentary lifestyle are some of the occupational hazards of adult life. Through the healing power of touch we can learn to take care of ourselves better. Taking the time to channel healing energy or enjoy a soothing foot massage can ease some of the day-to-day tensions of life and put us back in touch with ourselves and our priorities, to feel relaxed and at home in our bodies.

massage

Widely recognized as an effective method of holistic health care, massage is one of the oldest therapies in the world. It is based on manipulating the body's soft tissues with a few simple techniques.

HISTORY

For thousands of years some form of massage has been used to heal and soothe the sick. In ancient Greek and Roman times, massage was one of the principal methods of pain relief – Julius Caesar allegedly had daily treatments to ease his headaches and neuralgia. In the West, it seems to have

▾ REGULAR MASSAGE HELPS TO MAINTAIN THE COLLAGEN FIBRES, WHICH GIVE SKIN ITS ELASTICITY AND STRENGTH AND KEEP WRINKLES AT BAY.

played a vital role in health care until the Middle Ages, when it fell out of favour with the Catholic Church which regarded such contact as sinful. Its healing powers were rediscovered at the end of the 19th century by Professor Per Henrik Ling, a Swedish gymnast. Ling's methods formed the basis of modern massage – often referred to as Swedish massage. Support for this gentle, non-intrusive treatment has been growing ever since.

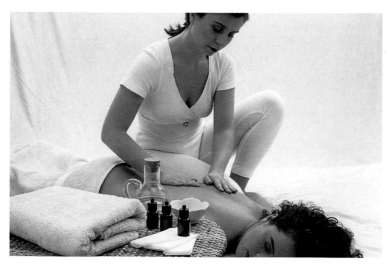

Healing Powers

Massage is primarily about touch. When used with skill and care, it can evoke many beneficial changes within the body, mind and spirit. Massage can ease pain and tension from stiff and aching muscles, boost a sluggish circulation, improve the health and appearance of the skin, help the body to eliminate toxins, support the immune system, encourage cellular renewal and aid digestion. As tense muscles relax, stiff joints loosen and nerves are soothed, inducing an all-over feeling of relaxation and wellbeing. Receiving a massage is a nourishing and calming experience that can increase self-confidence and self-esteem.

Applications

As a therapy, massage can help strains and sprains to heal more rapidly after injury and is generally useful for treating muscle and joint disorders such as arthritis and back pain. However, massage is probably most widely used in the treatment of stress-related disorders. If you are constantly exposed to the adverse effects of stress, it can lead to problems such as anxiety, depression, lethargy, insomnia, frequent tension headaches, hypertension, breathing problems and digestive disorders, for instance. While not a cure for specific complaints, the nurturing touch of another's hands helps soothe away mental stress and restores emotional equilibrium. There is also evidence to show that a massage treatment reduces the amount of stress hormones produced by the body, which can weaken the immune system. So, having a massage will help prevent as well as cure ill health.

▼ Everyone can benefit from the nurturing power of touch.

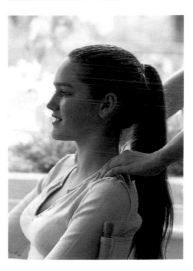

choosing massage oils

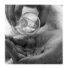

It is usual to work with oils when giving massage. The oil helps the hands to flow and glide over the body and it also lubricates the skin. There are many different types of oil to choose from.

VEGETABLE OILS

Probably the most popular and versatile massage oil is sweet almond. It is light, non-greasy and easily absorbed by the skin. Its neutral and non-allergenic properties make it suitable for all skin types – it may even be used on babies. Grapeseed oil seems to suit oily skins quite well, or soya oil is a useful alternative. Nut and seed oils are generally too rich and sticky to use on their own, but may be added to a lighter oil, such as almond, to create a mixture suitable for an individual skin type.

ESSENTIAL OILS

Fragrant essential oils have particular therapeutic properties, working on the mind and emotions as well as the physical body. They should never be used neat on the skin, but a few drops may be added to the

▼ MIX 5 DROPS OF ESSENTIAL OIL IN 10ML/ 2 TSP CARRIER OIL FOR A BODY MASSAGE.

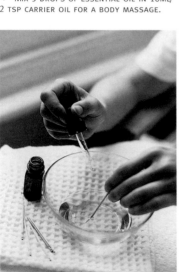

NUT & SEED OILS & THEIR USES

• Walnut: balances the nervous system; helpful for menstrual problems.
• Sesame: for treating stretch marks.
• Apricot kernel/peachnut/ evening primrose: all promote cellular regeneration; useful for facial massage.
• Hazelnut: for oily skin.
• Jojoba: for oily and sensitive skin; helpful for acne.
• Wheatgerm or avocado: for very dry skin.

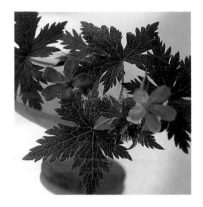

▲ A MASSAGE WITH GERANIUM OIL CAN HELP RELIEVE MOODINESS.

vegetable oil base mix (the "carrier"). You may blend up to three oils in any one treatment. Remember that essential oils are highly concentrated medicinal substances and should be handled with care. If in doubt, do not use them, and if any skin irritation occurs, wash the oil off with soap and warm water.

▼ ROSEMARY IS STIMULATING. IT CAN HELP RELIEVE DEPRESSION AND CLEAR THE MIND.

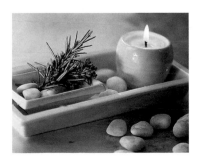

THE PROPERTIES & USES OF ESSENTIAL PLANT OILS

• Basil: useful as a massage for regulating the nervous system. It is a good tonic and stimulant, and helpful for muscle cramp.
• Camomile: relaxing; useful for tension headaches, inflamed skin conditions, menstrual problems and insomnia.
• Geranium: refreshing, anti-depressant; useful in blends; good for nervous tension and exhaustion.
• Juniper: uplifting, warming; primary use as a detoxifier, useful for treating cellulite. Avoid in pregnancy and if you suffer from kidney disease.
• Lavender: balancing, refreshing; one of the safest and most versatile of all essential oils; useful for tension headaches, stress and insomnia.
• Orange: refreshing, sedative; a tonic for anxiety and depression; useful for digestive problems.
• Rose: sedating, calming, anti-inflammatory, aphrodisiac; useful for muscular and nervous tension, dry, mature and aging skins.
• Rosemary: stimulating; useful for mental fatigue and debility. Avoid in pregnancy and with epilepsy.

preparing for massage

Giving and receiving massage is a relaxing and enjoyable experience. It is important to work in a supportive environment – one that is warm, quiet and draught-free – and to choose a time when you won't be disturbed.

FIRST STEPS

Begin by gathering together all the necessary equipment and materials. This will include massage oils, a selection of clean, soft towels, tissues and perhaps some candles and soft music to set the mood. Make sure the massage area is firm but comfortable; the floor or a futon padded with a thick layer of towels is fine, but an ordinary mattress is generally too soft and springy. It is best to wear comfortable loose-fitting clothes, to take off any jewellery and to make sure your nails are short. Do a few

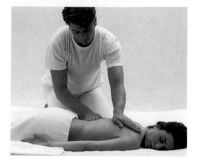

▲ A MASSAGE IS A RELAXING EXPERIENCE FOR THE RECIPIENT.

stretches and take some deep breaths to calm and centre yourself; giving a massage when you feel tense is counter-productive.

MAKING CONTACT

The initial contact is a key moment in massage. Gently place one hand on the top of the spine and the other near the base. When using oil, pour it on to your own hands first to warm it, never directly on to your partner's skin as cold oil can cause a shock and undo the relaxing effect. Using smooth, flowing strokes, spread the oil on to the skin then begin the massage.

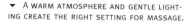

▼ A WARM ATMOSPHERE AND GENTLE LIGHTING CREATE THE RIGHT SETTING FOR MASSAGE.

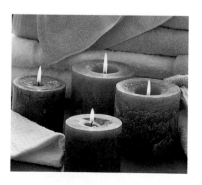

massage strokes

Massage techniques are relatively simple to learn. They range from a gentle, stroking action that relaxes the body to a more vigorous kneading, pummelling or hacking motion to stimulate and energize the system.

CIRCLING

This massage movement is useful for moving over large areas of muscle. The action releases areas of tension held in the muscles before deeper, stronger massage is used.

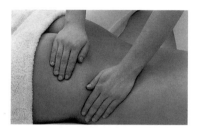

1 Lay both hands flat and parallel to each other about 10cm/4in apart. Circle both hands clockwise.

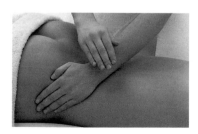

2 Lift up the right hand as it completes the first half-circle. Let the left hand pass underneath.

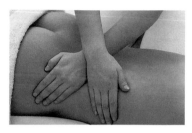

3 As the left hand continues to circle over the body, cross the right hand over it, dropping it lightly on the skin. Let the right hand form another half-circle before lifting off as the left hand completes its full circle. Repeat several times.

EFFLEURAGE

This technique describes long, soothing, stroking movements, using the flat of the hand (or fingers if you are working on small areas). These strokes are used at the beginning and end of the massage. They are also used in between other more stimulating strokes for continuity, and to establish contact with a new area of the body. They have a calming and reassuring effect and should be done slowly and gently.

▶

Petrissage

Kneading or petrissage movements stimulate the circulation and encourage the drainage of toxins. Generally, a single group of muscles or an individual muscle is worked on at a time. The basic kneading action is similar to kneading dough. Wringing movements also have a similar effect.

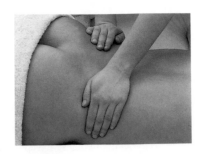

1 Place your right hand over the hip opposite to you and cup your left hand over the hip closest to you. Slide your hands towards each other with enough pressure to lift and roll the flesh on the sides of the body.

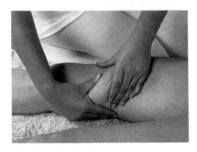

1 Grasp the flesh between fingers and thumb and push it towards the other hand. As you release the first hand, your second hand grasps the flesh and pushes it back towards the first hand. It is a continuous action, alternating the hands to squeeze and release.

Wringing

Like petrissage, wringing relies on the action of one hand pushing against the other to create a powerful squeezing action.

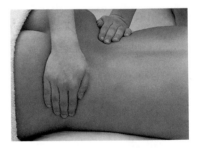

2 Decrease the pressure as you stroke across the back to your original position, hands passing each other to the opposite sides of the body. Without stopping, immediately begin to slide them back. Stroke your hands back and forth continuously while you wring up and down the lower back area.

FRICTION

Use friction techniques, such as pressure and knuckling, to work on specific areas of tightness and muscle spasm. Pressure techniques are less painful when performed along the direction of the muscle fibres.

1 To apply static pressure, press firmly into the muscle with the thumbs. Lean into the movement with the body, slowly deepening the pressure and then release.

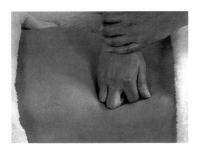

2 To release tension up the sides of the spine, use the knuckles in a loosely clenched fist on either side of the spine to produce rippling, circular movements.

CAUTION
Do not use tapotement on bony areas of the body. Never apply pressure on or below broken or varicose veins.

TAPOTEMENT

These movements are fast and stimulating, improving the circulation, and toning the skin and muscles. They are useful for working on fleshy areas of the body. Remember to keep your hands and wrists relaxed.

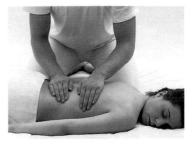

1 Cup the hands and make a brisk cupping action against a fleshy area, alternating the hands.

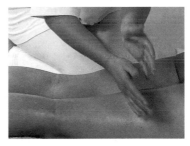

2 Use the outer edge of the palm and a chopping or hacking motion with alternate hands. Work rhythmically and rapidly.

shiatsu

The word shiatsu means "finger pressure" in Japanese. It is a method of holistic healing that is based on applying pressure to key points on the body. Unlike most other forms of bodywork, you remain fully clothed during treatment.

HISTORY

Shiatsu was developed in Japan in the early 20th century and has its roots in Traditional Chinese Medicine (TCM). A basic idea in TCM is the concept of the life force, known as "chi" in Chinese and "ki" in Japanese. The life force is the fundamental essence or spirit of life. Invisible like the air that we breathe, it is the energy that animates and nourishes all living things. Ki flows through the human body, circulating through the cells, tissues. muscles and internal organs, and influencing health and wellbeing on a physical, mental and emotional level.

YIN AND YANG

This energetic life force or ki is recognized as having two polar, yet complementary opposites called yin and yang.

◀ THE SYMBOL OF YIN YANG REPRESENTS BALANCING OPPOSITES.

Each of these represents different qualities: yin is feminine and passive, yang is masculine and active. The aim of shiatsu is to bring a harmony between the yin and yang energies of the body and its internal organs. This harmony can be disturbed through external trauma such as shock, or injury, or internal trauma such as depression or anxiety. This is when symptoms like aches and pains start to occur and

▼ BACKACHE IS JUST ONE OF MANY COMPLAINTS THAT CAN BE EASED WITH SHIATSU.

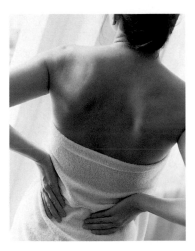

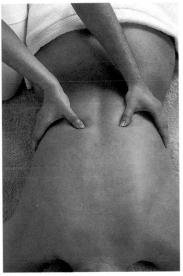

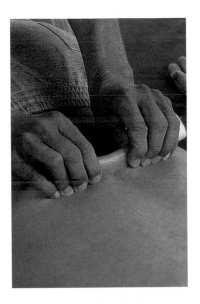

we start to experience a state of "dis-ease". In shiatsu, physical touch is used to assess the distribution of ki throughout the body and aims to correct any imbalances. This is done by applying pressure to specific points on the body where ki is concentrated, helping to release energy blocks and triggering the self-healing process.

BENEFITS

Shiatsu is particularly helpful for stress-related conditions, such as insomnia, tension headaches and digestive upsets, where the gentle, caring touch of another can help the

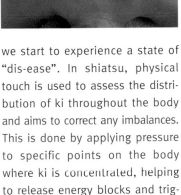

▲ ABOVE AND LEFT: TOUCH IS THE ESSENCE OF SHIATSU. A SHIATSU TREATMENT CAN CALM THE NERVOUS SYSTEM, STIMULATE THE CIRCULATION AND BOOST THE IMMUNE SYSTEM.

body to relax and unwind. It is also useful for improving the circulation and easing out stiffness in the muscles and joints. This makes it useful for treating conditions such as back pain, arthritis or asthma for instance. However, you do not need to be ill to enjoy the benefits of shiatsu. It works very well as a preventive system of health care; it helps to keep the energy flowing freely in the body and has a balancing effect on the body, mind and spirit.

the meridians

Vital energy "ki" flows through the body along invisible energy pathways, or meridians. These meridians connect all the different parts of the body together and for good health it is essential that this energy can flow freely along them.

BALANCE AND HEALTH

Rather like the veins and arteries of the physical body, the meridians conduct ki, the invisible "blood" of life, to and from the body's cells and organs, bringing nourishment and taking away poisons. If a meridian is blocked, it means that one part of the body is getting too much ki and enters a state of excess, or "jitsu", while another part is getting too little and becomes deficient, or "kyo". The system or organ of the body connected to this meridian is then thrown out of balance and begins to produce symptoms of "dis-ease".

Shiatsu recognizes that any symptoms, however small and insignificant they may appear, are a sign that the energy within the meridian system is out of balance. It is therefore important to deal with minor symptoms, as they may be an early warning of a more serious health condition that could develop if they go unchecked, or may develop into a health problem.

TSUBO

Along the meridians are highly charged energy points, known as "tsubo" in Japanese, or pressure points in English. By using different shiatsu techniques on these

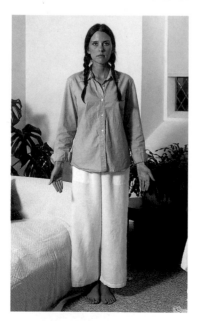

◀ THE MERIDIANS ARE ENERGY LINES RUN-NING THROUGH THE BODY. THEY ARE NOT VISIBLE TO THE EYE AND WILL NOT SHOW UP ON AN X-RAY.

points, such as pressure or stretching for instance, you can help to release any blocked ki and encourage the meridian to "open". This will allow excess ki to disperse or provide a boost where it is stagnant or depleted.

THE HARA

Ki enters the body through the breath, circulates through the meridians and is stored in the abdomen or "hara", at a special point approximately three finger-widths below the navel. This is the body's centre of gravity and the seat of vital energy. The level of energy in the hara can be used to diagnose and treat problems in all of the meridian lines.

THE TWELVE ORGANS

There are 12 main meridians, each of which is linked to an "organ" of the body. All the meridians either start or end in the hands or the feet and connect internally to the organ whose condition they reflect.

In shiatsu the organs of the body are perceived in a broader and less literal sense than in conventional thought. In Traditional Chinese Medicine (TCM), the body is seen as a kingdom with each organ having a governing role, an "official" responsible for different functions. When the officials work together and co-operate there is peace and harmony in the land (body). If there is disagreement or disorganization between the different officials, imbalances start to occur.

LUNG

Official function: jurisdiction.

Responsible for: the intake of fresh ki from the environment and the elimination of stagnant ki through exhalation.

Qualities: openness, positivity.

LARGE INTESTINE
Official function: elimination and exchange.
Responsible for: supporting the function of the lungs; the elimination of waste products from food, drink and stagnated ki.
Qualities: the ability to let go of clutter.

SPLEEN
Official function: storage.
Responsible for: general digestion of food and liquid; the flow of gastric juices and reproductive hormones; transformation and nourishment of the body.
Qualities: self-assurance and self-confidence.

STOMACH
Official function: in charge of the body's food store.
Responsible for: receiving and processing ingested food and drink; providing information for mental and physical nourishment.
Qualities: grounded, focused and reliable personality.

HEART
Official function: prime minister.
Responsible for: the blood and blood vessels; integrates external stimuli. The heart is the seat of the mind and emotions.
Qualities: joy, awareness and communication.

SMALL INTESTINE
Official function: treasurer.
Responsible for: converting food into energy; the quality of the blood and tissue reflects the condition of the small intestine.
Qualities: emotional stability, calm.

LUNG
HEART GOVERNOR
HEART

SMALL INTESTINE
TRIPLE HEATER
LARGE INTESTINE

LIVER
SPLEEN
KIDNEY

KIDNEY

Official function: energetic worker.
Responsible for: providing and storing ki for all other organs; governs reproduction, birth, growth and development; nourishes the spine, the bones and the brain.
Qualities: vitality, direction and willpower.

BLADDER

Official function: storage of overflow and fluid secretions.
Responsible for: purification and regulation.
Qualities: courage and the ability to move forward in life.

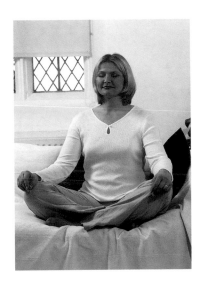

▲ TO EFFECTIVELY GIVE A HEALING TREATMENT YOU SHOULD FEEL CENTRED AND COMFORTABLE AND ATTUNED TO THE WORK IN HAND.

HEART GOVERNOR

Official function: joy and pleasure.
Responsible for: protecting the heart; is closely related to emotional responses.
Qualities: ability to influence relationships with others.

TRIPLE HEATER

Official function: plans construction.
Responsible for: transportation of energy, blood and heat to the peripheral parts of the body.
Qualities: helpful and emotionally interactive.

LIVER

Official function: planning.
Responsible for: storage of blood; ensures free flow of ki throughout the body.
Qualities: creative and full of ideas.

GALL BLADDER

Official function: decision making.
Responsible for: storing bile produced by the liver and distributing it to the small intestine.
Qualities: practical; ability to turn ideas into reality.

basic shiatsu techniques

Shiatsu uses the hands, elbows, knees and feet to apply pressure on specific meridian points. It can also incorporate passive stretching movements to help to loosen the body, manipulate the joints and ease tension.

FIRM PRESSURE

When giving a shiatsu treatment, focus on your breathing and posture. All movement should emanate from the hara (abdomen); this brings a calm, meditative quality to the mind and will be relayed through your healing touch. When applying pressure, lean on the appropriate point for up to 10 seconds before slowly releasing the pressure.

THUMB PRESSURE

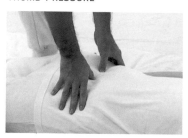

The bladder meridian is the largest and runs down each side of the spine to the sacrum (the triangular bone forming the back of the pelvis). A steady thumb pressure applied on the sacral points can relieve sciatica and lower-back pain.

PALM PRESSURE

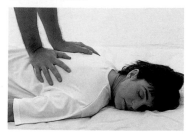

Relax and open out the hands. Shift your weight into the palms and heels of the hands to press firmly but gently along the bladder meridian points.

STRETCHING

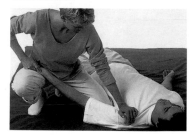

Gentle stretches along the meridians help the body. The practitioner opens the chest by gently stretching the lung meridian in the arm.

Do-in

This self-massage technique is designed to improve the circulation and flow of ki through the body. It will wake up your brain and aid concentration and mental clarity.

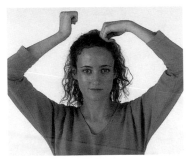

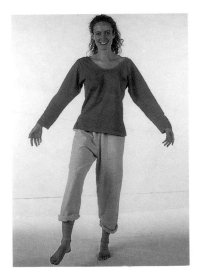

1 Shake your arms, hands, legs and feet, letting go of tension. Breathe deeply, keeping your back straight.

CAUTION
Seek the advice of a qualified practitioner if you suffer from high blood pressure, varicose veins, osteoporosis, thrombosis, epilepsy, if you are pregnant, or suffer from serious illnesses.

2 Make a loose fist with both hands. Keep your wrists relaxed and gently tap the top of your head with your fingers or knuckles. Adjust the pressure as needed and use your fingertips or palms for lighter stimulation. Work your way all around the head, covering the sides, front and back.

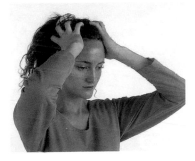

3 Finish by pulling your fingers through your hair a few times. This stimulates the bladder and gall bladder meridians that run across the top and side of your head.

reflexology

The word "reflex" means to reflect. In reflexology, specific points on the hands or feet reflect another part of the body. By working on these points you can treat health problems elsewhere in the body-mind system.

HISTORY

Foot and hand treatments have been used in healing traditions across the world for thousands of years, but reflexology in its present form is a relatively recent discovery. In the early 20th century, an American doctor, William Fitzgerald, found that applying pressure to points on the hands or feet could help to relieve pain elsewhere in the body. Eunice Ingham, a physiotherapist, went on to map out these pressure points or reflex zones, matching up areas of the body with specific points on the feet and hands. Later, people discovered that these points also relate to certain emotional and psychological states.

BALANCING THE BODY

Reflexology is based on two important principles: that small parts of the body can be used to treat the whole, and that the body has the ability to heal itself. As a result of illness, stress or injury, the body's systems are thrown out of balance and its vital energy path-

▼ REFLEXOLOGY CAN BE PRACTISED ANY-WHERE FOR RELAXATION AND HEALTH.

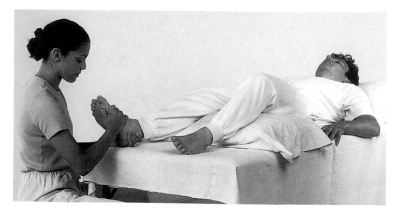

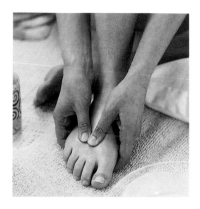

▲ YOU CAN PRACTISE THE HEALING EFFECTS OF REFLEXOLOGY ON YOURSELF.

TREATMENT

Reflexology is becoming widely recognized as an effective treatment for many health problems. It works well for any condition involving congestion and/or inflammation, such as sinus problems, digestive disturbances, menstrual problems or eczema. It is also an effective method of pain relief and is useful for treating back pain, rheumatism, arthritis or headaches, for instance. A reflexology treatment is relaxing, making it popular for treating stress-related disorders, calming anxiety, alleviating tension and encouraging restful sleep. Many people enjoy reflexology because of its "feel good" factor.

ways are blocked. Messages between the brain and nervous system become distorted and the body begins to produce distress signals or symptoms in its call for help. These symptoms of "dis-ease" will show up in various ways (such as headaches or mood swings for instance) and toxic waste matter accumulates around the relevant reflex points. Places on the feet where there are toxic deposits will feel tender, sensitive or painful; or they may feel hard, tight or lumpy, or like little grains. Stimulating these points with massage helps the congestion to disperse and frees up energy blocks elsewhere in the system, encouraging the body to rebalance.

▼ REFLEXOLOGISTS REGARD THE FEET AS A MAP OF THE WHOLE BODY.

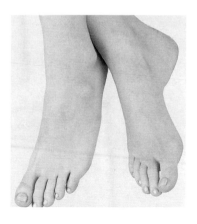

reflex zones

In reflexology the fingers are used to apply pressure-point therapy to certain key points on the feet and/or hands. These points, known as reflex zones, are linked to the body's internal organs and systems and its external structure.

ENERGY CHANNELS

The body is divided into ten vertical energy zones that run from the head to reflex points on the hands and feet, five on the left, five on the right. These zones are similar to the meridians used in shiatsu. All parts of the body that fall into a particular zone are linked by nerve pathways and mirrored in a corresponding reflex point on the hands or feet.

If there is any imbalance within a zone, the body can produce a range of symptoms that relate to several different body parts that all fall within that zone. Problems with the eyes for instance may indicate an underlying problem with the kidneys. A reflexology treatment, therefore, would not only work on the reflex point related to the eyes, but would also treat the kidneys and any other relevant parts of the body in zone two.

CROSS REFLEXES

Reflexology also works with cross reflexes. Parts of the upper body correspond to parts of the lower body, so that the arms correspond to the legs (the elbows with the knees, the wrists with the ankles), the hips with the shoulders and the hands with the feet. This is useful when an area of the body is too painful to work on directly; for instance, to treat a dislocated right shoulder you can work on the reflex for the right hip.

ZONES ON THE FEET

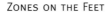

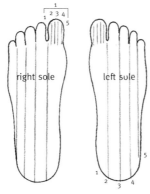

right sole left sole

◀ LOOKING AT THE SOLES OF THE FEET, THE RIGHT SIDE OF YOUR BODY IS REPRESENTED BY YOUR RIGHT FOOT AND THE LEFT SIDE BY YOUR LEFT FOOT.

Zones on the Body

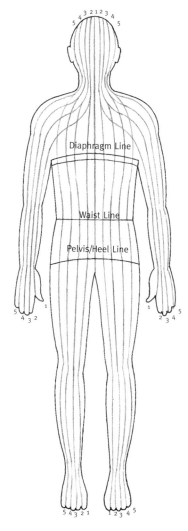

Diaphragm Line

Waist Line

Pelvis/Heel Line

▲ THE ZONES RUN VERTICALLY THROUGH THE BODY FROM HEAD TO FEET AND HANDS.

Parts of the Body

Both feet together hold the reflexes to the whole body. It can be helpful to divide the body into different areas, tying these in with the relevant zones of the feet. Working from head to foot:

• The head and neck are represented by the toes: the right side of the head with the right big toe, and the left side with the left big toe. The eight little toes represent specific parts of the head, such as eyes, ears, mouth and so on. The kidneys and the eyes are both linked by the energy in zone two.

• The lungs, chest and shoulder areas are represented by the balls of the feet.

• The abdomen is represented by the area from the balls of the feet to the middle of the arch.

• The pelvic area is represented by the soles and sides of the heels and across the top of the ankle.

• The spine is represented by the line that runs along the inner edge of the feet.

• The limbs are represented on the outer edge of the feet, working from the toes to the heels are the arms, shoulders, hips, legs, knees and lower back.

a mirror of the body

The feet are believed to mirror the shape of the body, with the organs and body parts appearing in roughly the same position as they occur in the body. Each foot represents the left- and right-hand side of the body.

FOOT CHARTS

When you find a tender or congested part of the foot, you may look for that part on the charts and see approximately which reflex the tenderness lies on. However, picking out certain reflexes in isolation is only really effective in the context of working on the whole foot. Remember also that the charts are only guidelines for interpretation. Every pair of feet will be different and in reality your organs overlap each other, so everything will not "fit" neatly in exactly the same area as shown on the chart.

THE SPINE

Both feet together hold the reflexes to the whole body. The part that holds the spine therefore runs down the medial line along the inner edge of each foot. The spinal reflex is particularly important. It should always be massaged and the reflex worked thoroughly. The spinal column is not only our main bony support, but it also contains

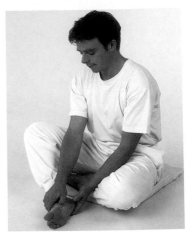

▲ YOU CAN TREAT YOUR OWN AILMENTS WITH REFLEXOLOGY.

the spinal cord, the central energy channel that transmits messages to and from the brain through the central nervous system.

PEDI-CURE

There are more than 70,000 nerve endings on the sole of each foot. By stimulating specific points on the feet, information is transmitted via the nervous system to the brain and a healing process is triggered.

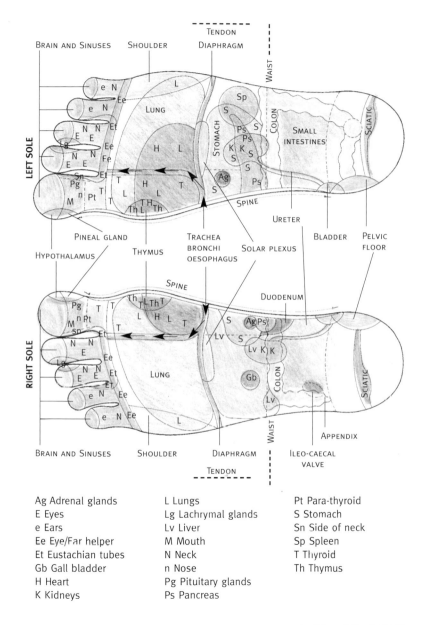

Ag Adrenal glands	L Lungs	Pt Para-thyroid
E Eyes	Lg Lachrymal glands	S Stomach
e Ears	Lv Liver	Sn Side of neck
Ee Eye/Ear helper	M Mouth	Sp Spleen
Et Eustachian tubes	N Neck	T Thyroid
Gb Gall bladder	n Nose	Th Thymus
H Heart	Pg Pituitary glands	
K Kidneys	Ps Pancreas	

basic reflexology techniques

Applying thumb and/or finger pressure to the reflex points on the feet helps to release congestion and stimulates healing. There are several basic techniques which are simple to learn. The movements should be small and controlled.

HOLDING AND SUPPORT
When you practise any technique, always make sure that the hand or foot you are working on is secure. It will mean your partner will be more relaxed and you can work much more effectively.

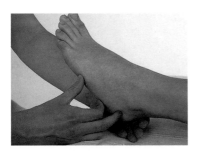

1 Use one hand to hold the foot and the other to work on it. Position your holding hand near the working hand, not at the other end of the foot as this can feel insecure.

THUMB WALKING
This is the most common method and a useful technique to use all over the foot. It is done with the pad of the thumb that "walks" forward in caterpillar-like movements.

Use one hand only, the other holds and supports the foot or hand you are working on.

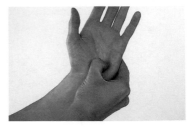

1 Press the thumb of one of your hands down on the skin of the other hand using a firm pressure.

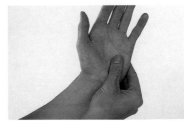

2 Ease off the pressure and slide or skate forward as you straighten your thumb in a caterpillar movement. Stop and press again. Keep your movements slow, continuous and rhythmic.

Finger Walking

This technique uses the fingers and is useful for bony areas.

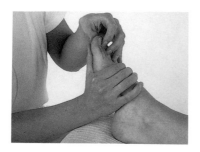

1 Hold the foot or hand with your right hand and fingerwalk from the tip of the big toe with your left index finger.

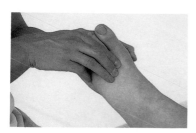

2 Firmly hold the foot or hand with one hand and fingerwalk down the top of the foot towards the toes, using the three middle fingers of the other hand together. This area can be very sensitive so take care not to press too hard with the fingers. Try to keep the pressure firm and even, but comfortable.

Rotating

This technique is good for tender reflexes, or for when you want to work on a specific small point. Vary the pressure as is comfortable.

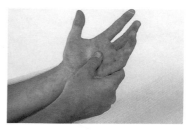

Using a firm pressure, press and rotate the thumb into the point.

Pinpointing

Use this technique for deep or less accessible reflexes. Restrict it to the fleshy, padded parts of the feet as it can be quite painful.

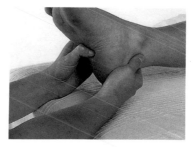

Supporting the heel, press deeply into the tissues with the inner corner of your thumb.

reiki

Channelling divine or cosmic healing energy through the hands is one of the oldest and most profound methods of healing known. Reiki is a special technique that brings the ability to heal within the grasp of everyone.

HISTORY

Reiki (pronounced ray-key) means universal ("rei") life force ("ki") in Japanese. With its roots in Tibetan Buddhism, the ancient healing methods of reiki were rediscovered in the 19th century by Dr Mikao Usui, a Japanese mystic, during a vision. These methods were regarded as sacred knowledge, and the secrets were passed down from master to student in special initiation ceremonies. Today the tradition of master and student continues, and reiki practitioners have been through special "attunements" with a modern-day master to receive this ancient knowledge and open up a healing channel. It is relatively easy to find a reiki master and become a reiki initiate, but it is possible for anyone to channel healing reiki energy by understanding and applying a few basic principles.

UNIVERSAL LAW

Reiki is about tuning in to the laws of the universe and working in harmony with them. The universe is a place of boundless energy that flows through space and time, and through everything here on Earth. We are not separate, isolated identities but connected to the universe and everything in it by this cosmic energy, the breath of life that nurtures and sustains us. This energy is sometimes known as the

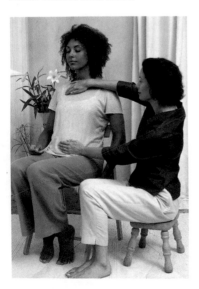

▼ A REIKI PRACTITIONER CHANNELS HEALING ENERGY THROUGH THEIR HANDS.

life force and its healing power is love. It is a force for good in the world that transcends time and place, colour and creed, and any negative, destructive impulses that threaten the health and wellbeing of life. Reiki invites us to open up and trust in this great love, allowing it to flow through us, bringing positive healing wherever it is needed. We can channel this healing energy for the benefit of ourselves and other people, as well as to treat plants, animals and even places.

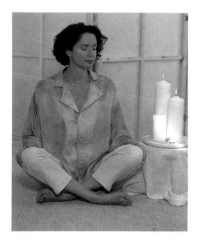

▲ WE CAN ALL BENEFIT FROM REIKI AND EACH OF US CAN CHANNEL REIKI ENERGY.

▼ REIKI CHANNELS THE ESSENTIAL ENERGY OF THE UNIVERSE TO CREATE WELLBEING.

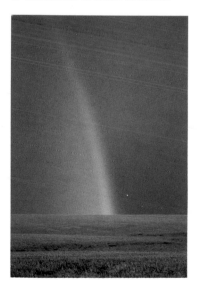

BENEFITS

Giving and receiving reiki is a relaxing experience. It is particularly effective for calming and soothing negative emotional states, for relieving pain and for treating stress-related conditions, such as insomnia, fatigue or tension headaches, for instance. A reiki treatment helps to rebalance the body's energy systems and generally promotes good health and wellbeing. Done regularly it can help to protect the body against illness and negative influences as it helps to realign the human energy system with the healing vibrations of love and light.

subtle anatomy

There is much more to the human body than meets the eye. Invisible energy centres, or chakras, run up the body from the base of the spine to the crown of the head. The chakras are widely used in reiki healing.

WHEELS OF ENERGY

The chakra system has been used in the East for thousands of years. The word "chakra" means wheel in the Sanskrit language, and a chakra may be thought of as a spinning vortex of energy, a wheel of light. There are seven of these energy centres, each vibrating at a different frequency, from the lowest at the base rising to the highest at the crown. Each of the chakras governs a particular area of the body and is associated with certain characteristics (see table).

▼ THE CHAKRAS ARE VORTICES OR INVISIBLE WHEELS OF ENERGY.

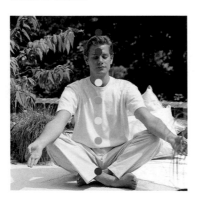

THE ENDOCRINE SYSTEM

The chakras act in perfect synchronicity with the endocrine system. This amazing system controls the functions of the body at a cellular level through seven major glands in the body, each of which is associated with a particular chakra. The glands of the endocrine system are responsible for the correct amount of chemical nutrients, or hormones, fed to each of our organs, and if one of them has an imbalance it can be felt in the chakra.

HEALTH AND THE CHAKRAS

The chakras are connected to each other and every part of the body by fine energy channels, called "nadis". For health and wellbeing, energy should be able to circulate freely through the nadis and the chakra system. Blocked or excess energy in any part of this energy circuit will create health problems on a physical, mental or emotional level. The longer this is left

THE SEVEN CHAKRAS

chakra	colour	governs	concerned with
1st root, at the base of the spine.	red	gonads/ovaries, skeletal structure, large intestine and lower body.	physical survival, energy distribution, ambition, security, practicality.
2nd hara, just below the navel.	orange	bladder and circulation.	sexuality, creativity, feelings, emotions and pleasure.
3rd solar plexus, just below the ribcage.	yellow	adrenal glands, spleen, pancreas, stomach.	identity, self-confidence, personal power, desires and wishes.
4th heart, in the centre of the chest.	green	thymus gland, immune system, lungs.	relationships, personal development, compassion, self-acceptance, aesthetic impulse.
5th throat.	blue/ turquoise	thyroid gland, lymphatic, immune and neurological systems.	self-expression, communication, trust.
6th "third eye", at the centre of the brow.	indigo	pituitary gland, central nervous system.	understanding, perception, intuition, clarity and insight, spiritual knowing, psychic abilities.
7th crown, at or just above the top of the head.	violet	pineal gland, ancient mammalian brain.	openness, connection to higher energies and spiritual realms, self-realization. Maintains overall balance of the chakra system.

untreated, the more complex the problem that is likely to develop will be. Reiki teaches us to become more attuned to our bodies. The treatments can be used to unblock and rebalance the energy in the chakras, which can be felt by your hands as balls of energy.

reiki hand positions

In a reiki treatment, the hands are positioned at various places on the body. In order for the energy flow to be focused, the fingers and thumbs are held together, and the hands kept flat or very slightly cupped.

If you have not been officially attuned to reiki, prepare yourself at a quiet time, when your attention can be fully attuned to yourself. Visualize a stream of golden healing light entering your body through the crown chakra. See yourself as an open and receptive channel for this energy, allowing it to enter and pass through your body via the hands, on to the body of your partner.

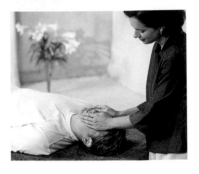

1 Place the hands over the eyes. This position aids clear vision and energizes the eyes.

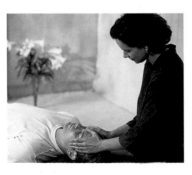

2 Slide the hands sideways on to the temples. This position helps to dispel tension in the face.

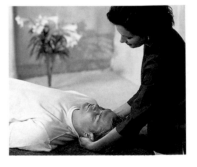

3 Bring your hands round to underneath your partner's head, just above the neck so that you are cradling it. This position balances the energy in both sides of the brain and releases mental tension.

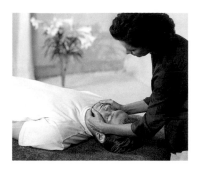

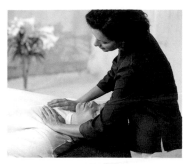

4 Remove your hands and place them with the heels of the palms on the side of the neck and with the palms and fingers lightly on the throat. This can help to release emotional trauma and upset.

5 Slide the hands on to the top of the chest. This position is relaxing and reassuring. Move to one side and continue down the trunk, placing your hands in a straight line across the chakra points.

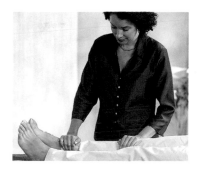

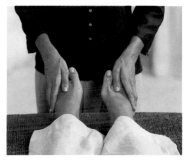

6 Continue working down, first one leg and then the other in as many stages as feels right. Working along the legs and channelling healing energy helps to balance and relax the recipient's lower body.

7 To finish, stand at the foot of your partner and finish by placing the hands on the feet, first the upper feet, then the soles. This helps to "ground" the energy so that your partner doesn't feel too floaty or light-headed at the end of the treatment.

self-treatment with reiki

It is a good idea to practise reiki on yourself. This will increase your self-confidence when giving treatments to other people, as you will have experienced its healing powers first hand. It will also nourish and refresh you.

REIKI SELF-TREATMENT

You can give reiki to yourself at any time of the day. Some people like to start with it first thing in the morning in preparation for the day ahead. Others find it helpful to end the day with reiki, helping the body to relax and unwind in preparation for sleep. Ideally, it is best to set aside a full hour for a reiki self-treatment, but if this is not possible, 10–15 minutes set aside on a regular basis will bring good results and a healthier outlook.

Either sit in a comfortable upright position or lie down where you won't be disturbed. Set your alarm clock if you have appointments, and unplug the telephone. Close your eyes and centre yourself by breathing gently into the abdomen. Take in a deep breath, hold for a few moments and exhale. Repeat this a few times.

Imagine that golden, healing reiki energy is flowing into your body, circulating along the subtle energy pathways, nourishing every

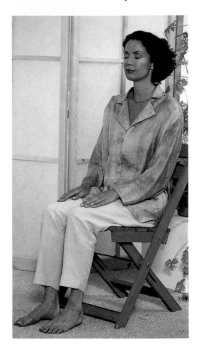

▲ A REIKI SELF-TREATMENT WILL LEAVE YOU FEELING REFRESHED AND READY FOR THE DAY.

cell and organ. Place your hands on any areas of your body that you feel need particular attention. Leave them there for as long as is comfortable. You may notice that the area of your body becomes warm as the energy circulates.

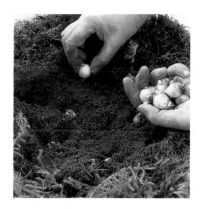

▲ THE FLOWERS, SHRUBS, EVEN BULBS IN YOUR GARDEN WILL BENEFIT FROM REIKI.

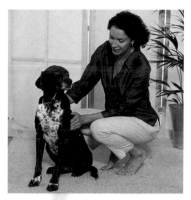

▲ PETS CAN BENEFIT FROM REIKI TOO — USE IT TO MAINTAIN GENERAL HEALTH.

REIKI ANYWHERE

Remember that there is nothing for your brain to "learn" with reiki. It is a question of being open to its healing powers and willing to let the energy flow through you. Cultivate the reiki habit and bring reiki treatments into other activities. Try relaxing back in a warm bath, and practise the hand positions on your face and torso. Reiki can be worked into a foot massage or a beauty treatment, or if you have a busy day, give yourself reiki as you go along. This can be done while watching television, queuing at the supermarket checkout or sitting in a traffic jam, for instance. Just put your palms anywhere on your body, imagine the healing energy entering you and say to yourself, "Reiki flow!" You will soon feel the benefits.

▼ GREETING THE DAY WITH A SALUTE TO THE SUN: ADDING AN ELEMENT OF RITUAL TO YOUR MORNING ROUTINE WILL CREATE A HAPPY DAY.

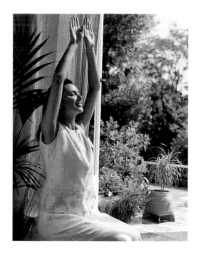

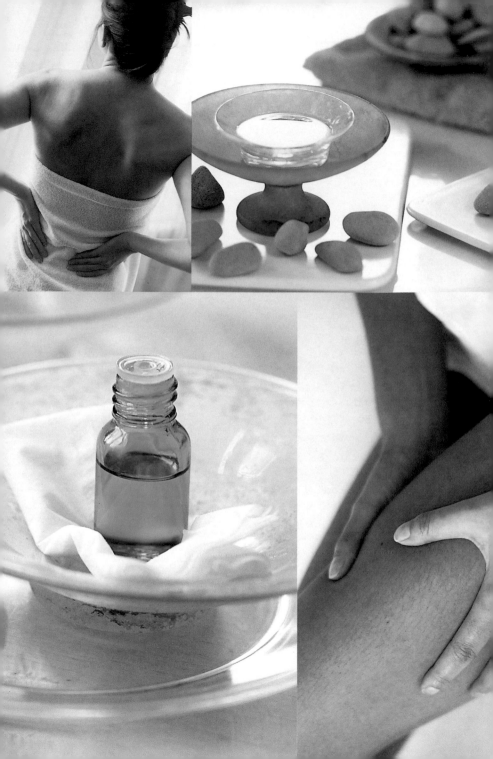

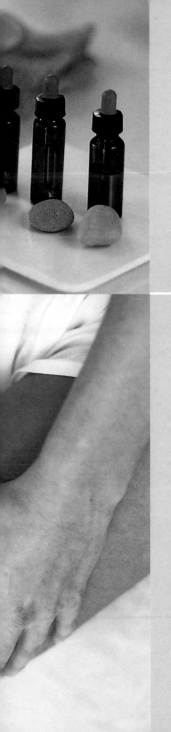

the healing touch

Many common health problems are related to stress and lifestyle. When we feel overwhelmed and unable to cope, the body's fine-tuning is knocked off balance and things start to go awry. The body produces a range of annoying and unpleasant symptoms. Many of these minor ailments respond well to the healing touch of massage, reflexology, reiki and/or shiatsu.

The following pages include step-by-step sequences and useful tips to treat a range of minor complaints, including backache, tension headaches, muscle pain, fluid retention and repetitive strain injuries. There are also treatments designed to improve the circulation and digestion, to relieve stress and tension and to enhance the quality of sleep. Some of these treatments can be practised on yourself, while others need a partner. They can all be done in comfort and safety at home.

backaches

More working days are lost through backache than from any other cause. Common causes of backache include poor posture, injury through straining and lifting, pregnancy, stress and muscular tension.

Back pain can vary from a dull, persistent, nagging ache to a sharp, searing pain. Tightness in the muscles around the spinal cord constricts the body's main energy pathway, affecting the central nervous system. The pain itself is also very draining. The soothing touch of another's hands can be very healing; reflexology and reiki are both helpful.

REFLEXOLOGY RELIEVER
A simple but effective reflexology treatment can help to release tension and relax the supporting muscles. The inside edge of the foot represents the spine.

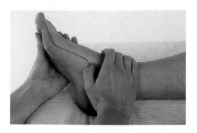

1 Thumbwalk along the spine, supporting the outer edge of the foot.

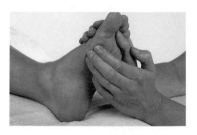

2 Fingerwalk across the spinal reflex, right down the instep, in stripes.

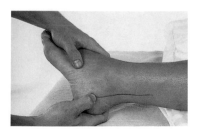

3 Thumbwalk up the helper reflexes.

TIPS FOR AVOIDING BACK PAIN
• Improve your posture; don't slump but sit straight, make sure your chair supports you.
• Take regular, gentle exercise, such as swimming or yoga.
• Invest in a firm mattress.
• Bend from the hips and knees when lifting heavy objects.

REIKI RELAXER

A gentle reiki treatment is another way of helping the body to relax. It can also address the underlying emotional and mental state that may be contributing to the problem. For instance, backache is often caused by worrying and feeling burdened. Lower back pain is linked to problems in the first chakra, indicating insecurity in material matters – such as worry about money.

Your partner should be sitting upright on a backless chair, or lying face down on the floor.

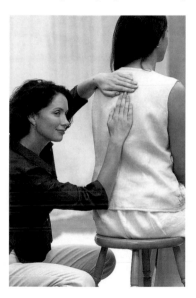 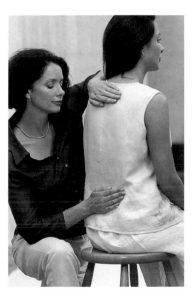

1 Place your hands in the shape of a T-cross between the shoulder blades and down the spine. This position treats the upper back and shoulder areas, stimulating the heart chakra and surrounding organs. Concentrate on the healing energy of your touch.

2 Allow your hands to be drawn to any other areas of the back where healing is needed. Finish by placing your hands at the top and bottom of the spine in the "spirit level" position, to balance the energy along the backbone and through the chakras.

headaches

The majority of "everyday" headaches are caused by stress and tension. Other common triggers include eyestrain, hangovers, lack of sleep and exercise, caffeine overload, missed meals and hormonal swings.

REFLEXOLOGY FOR HEADACHES
A foot treatment can work wonders on a tension headache. Headaches generally mean there is too much energy in the head and eyes, caused by excessive worry, mental work or eyestrain for instance. Reflexology can help to release the energy, encouraging it to disperse through the rest of the body.

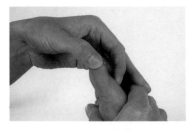

1 For pain relief, work the hypothalamus reflex. This controls the release of endorphins.

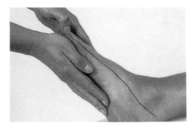

2 Work down the spine to take pressure away from the head. This will draw energy down the body.

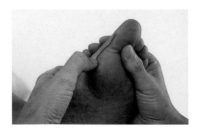

3 Work the cervical spine on the big toe. Work the neck of all the toes to relieve tension.

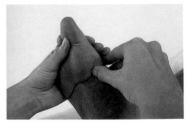

4 When we are tense our breathing is tight and shallow. Work the diaphragm area to encourage the breathing to become deeper.

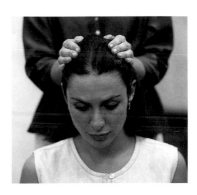

REIKI HEADACHE SOOTHER

A reiki treatment can help to melt away tensions and restore peace and equilibrium. It is best if your partner sits upright for this treatment, although it can also be done with him or her lying down.

1 Place your hands on each side of the head at the back cupping the skull. This helps to dispel tension rising from the neck and balances energy in the brain.

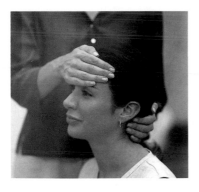

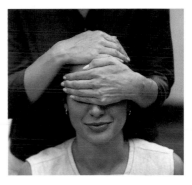

2 Place one hand on the forehead and the other at the base of the skull, cradling the head firmly in your hand.

3 Finish by gently placing one hand across the brow, covering the eyes. Place the other hand on top of the head, touching the first hand. Hold the position firmly. This position helps relieve emotional stress and is soothing for the recipient.

muscle pain & cramp

Muscles are the body's connecting tissue; their elasticity enables us to move. Pain in the muscles may result from injury or from overuse. Cramps are painful, involuntary muscle spasms.

MUSCLE RELAXING REFLEXOLOGY Reflexology can help to reduce inflammation and pain in the muscles and nerve endings. It can also relax muscle spasm. Before concentrating on the specific area of pain, work the hypothalamus reflex first to help with pain relief.

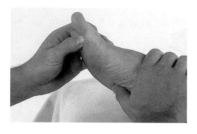

1 Work the adrenal gland reflexes on both feet thoroughly. These glands deal with inflammation and aid good muscle tone when working effectively.

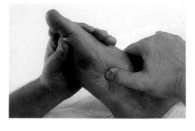

2 Thumbwalk along the spine to treat the central nervous system in the spinal cord.

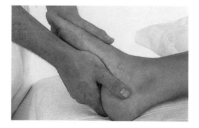

3 To ease cramp, hold the foot and massage the appropriate reflex using the foot chart as a guide.

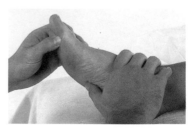

4 Work the parathyroid reflexes round the neck of the big toe.

MASSAGE FOR CALF CRAMP

Calf cramp can be triggered by exercise, repetitive action or sitting awkwardly. Cramp may indicate poor circulation or a deficiency of calcium or salt. Massage improves the circulation and alleviates pain. It also helps eliminate lactic acid, a waste product stored in the muscle tissue after exercise.

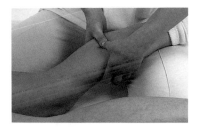

1 Apply thumb pressure into the cramped muscle for 8–10 seconds.

2 Work from the ankle to the thigh using long effleurage strokes.

HAMSTRING CRAMP MASSAGE

It is usually underused or ill-prepared muscles that go into cramp during exercise.

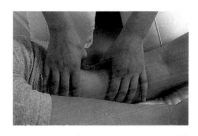
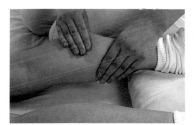

1 Raise the ankle on a small pillow and begin by massaging the back of the thigh using alternate hands in slow, rhythmical stroking movements. Then apply static pressure to the middle of the thigh with the thumbs, holding for 8–10 seconds.

2 Firmly knead the calf muscle. Squeeze, press and release the muscle using one hand after the other. Finish the massage by doing some soothing effleurage strokes up from ankle to thigh and back down again.

tennis elbow & repetitive strain

 Overuse of any part of the body puts a strain on the muscles and tendons and can result in painful conditions, such as tennis elbow or repetitive strain injury (RSI). Both of these conditions can be helped with touch therapies.

TENNIS ELBOW MASSAGE
Inflammation of the tendon running along the forearm to the elbow creates pain. Sportspeople and gardeners are particularly at risk. Massage can help to ease the pain.

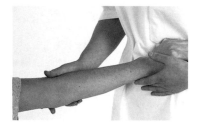

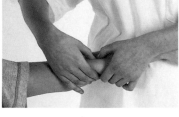

1 Support your partner's wrist in one hand and use soothing strokes along both sides of the arm from the wrist to the elbow and back again. Repeat several times.

2 Rest the hand against your side. Work up the arm, from wrist to elbow and back, making small circular movements.

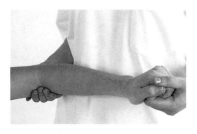

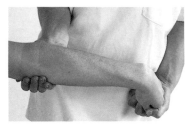

3 Stand to one side of your partner, secure their hand in yours and support their elbow with your other hand. Flex the elbow forward.

4 Bring the hand back to give the tendons that are attached to the bones a good stretch.

REFLEXOLOGY FOR REPETITIVE STRAIN
Repetitive strain can affect any part of the body that is overused. It is an occupational hazard for keyboard operators, where a stiff neck and shoulders, aching wrists and pain and weakness in the forearm are increasingly common problems. Reflexology can help to ease some of the discomfort.

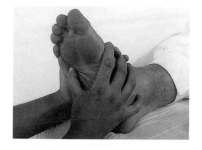

1 Work the shoulder reflexes thoroughly by using the thumbwalking technique. Gently fingerwalk across the same area on the top of the foot, with the three middle fingers held together.

TIPS FOR KEYBOARD WORKERS
• Make sure your wrist is well supported. Mouse mats are available with inbuilt wrist supports.
• Take regular breaks away from the keyboard.
• Flex and rotate the fingers and wrists, to keep them supple and stop them from aching.
• Massage hands and forearms on a regular basis.

2 Rotate the ankles to ease aching wrists and stimulate healing within the joints. Work down the outside of the foot to relax the shoulders and arms.

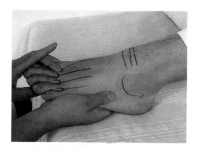

3 Work the lymph system on both feet to encourage toxins to drain away. Fingerwalk down the lines from the toes towards the ankle, then work around the ankle.

fluid retention & menstrual issues

 A heavy feeling in the legs and puffy, swollen ankles are typical signs of fluid retention. The problem is often aggravated by hot weather, prolonged periods of standing, premenstrual tension, long haul flights and pregnancy.

MASSAGE TO IMPROVE CIRCULATION
Excess fluid indicates that the kidneys and/or circulation are not working properly. Massaging the legs and the thighs will improve the local circulation and so bring more blood and oxygen to the muscles. Firm effleurage movements are particularly helpful. They should always be done in one direction, towards the heart.

TIPS TO AVOID FLUID RETENTION
• Drink plenty of water to help the kidneys flush out (at least six glasses a day).
• Remember to increase your water intake in hot weather.
• Include raw food in your diet.
• Regular massage will improve the circulation and drainage of toxins.
• Avoid prolonged sitting or standing in one spot.

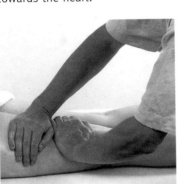

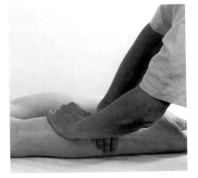

1 Place your hands on your partner's thigh and stroke upwards to the buttock several times using smooth effleurage strokes. Keep the pressure light but steady, letting one hand follow the other.

2 Move your hands down to the calf and stroke up to the back of the knee a few times. Repeat these two steps, always starting the massage on the upper leg and always stroking towards the heart.

Shiatsu Menstrual Treatment

Used on the feet, shiatsu can help to stimulate the body's energy system, improving circulation and the drainage of toxins. There are also specific points that can help with menstrual problems.

1 With a loose fist, tap the sole of the foot. Then gently massage the whole foot thoroughly with both hands.

2 Massage the web between each toe and then massage the toe joints. The point between the big toe and the second toe is good for period pains (do not use this massage during pregnancy).

3 Come to the sole of your foot and apply pressure to it with your thumb. This will have a revitalizing effect upon your body and stimulate energy flow.

4 Use your thumbs to massage the area under the ankle bone. This is a good point to use for any menstrual disorders. Use your thumb and press firmly.

▶ Instead of suffering from period pains, try a shiatsu self-treatment.

Useful Aromatic Oils

- Pine: reducing puffiness in the legs, particularly after prolonged standing and in late pregnancy.
- Geranium, juniper, rosemary: premenstrual fluid retention.
- Fennel, juniper, lemon: detoxifying oils.
- Cypress, geranium, pine: after long-haul flights.

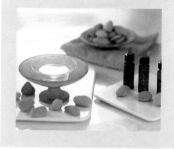

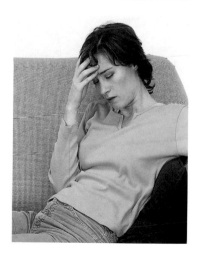

improving circulation

The circulatory system connects all the systems of the body. Its tone and vitality is fundamental to life and to the integration of the whole body. There are many steps we can take to help it function effectively.

HAND AND FOOT MASSAGE

Cold feet and hands are a sign of poor circulation. When we breathe in, oxygen from the air is absorbed into the blood and carried to the heart. It travels around the body, carrying vital nutrients to every cell and returning waste products for disposal. Poor circulation means that the body's tissues and organs are inadequately nourished and that toxins are not removed properly, leading to many other health problems. A massage will help to warm hands and feet, and improve the circulation.

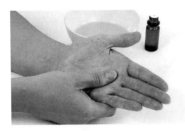

1 Using a little oil, massage the palm of the hand with a steady, circular movement of the thumb.

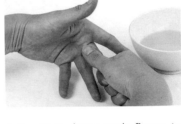

2 Squeeze down each finger to stretch and loosen the joints, pushing towards the palm. Repeat.

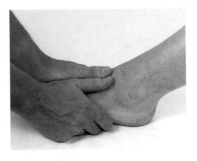

◂ **3** To stretch the foot, use both hands with the thumbs on top and fingers underneath the foot. Keep a loose but firm grip. Move the thumbs outward, as if breaking a piece of bread. Repeat several times, keeping the fingers still while moving your thumbs.

Shiatsu Techniques

Working a shiatsu treatment on each side of the spine is invigorating and relaxing. Rubbing and rolling techniques are useful for improving the circulation – of both blood and energy – throughout the whole body.

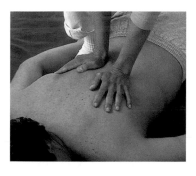

1 Use the palms to apply gentle but firm pressure down each side of the spine.

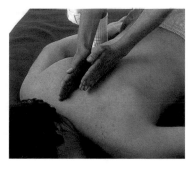

2 Using the side of your hands, vigorously rub down each side of the spine a few times.

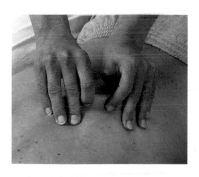

3 Pinch and take hold of the skin on the lower part of the spine. Lift the tissue and gradually roll it up the spine. Roll the skin from the spine, out towards the sides to cover the entire back.

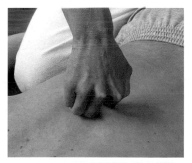

4 Use your index and middle fingers to pinch and take hold of the tissue. Twist and lift the skin at the same time. Work within your partner's pain threshold. Cover the whole back using this technique.

improving digestion

If we are what we eat, then the healthy functioning of the digestive system is essential. Stress and tension are responsible for many digestive disturbances, including bloating, constipation, abdominal cramps, diarrohea and indigestion.

SHIATSU TREATMENTS

In shiatsu, the Stomach meridian is vital for the production of "ki" in the body. These movements help to relax the body and ease any digestive disturbances.

▸ **1** Sit at your partner's side and place your right hand on the stomach. Note the breathing rate: fast and shallow indicates tension. When you are attuned to your partner's breathing, continue.

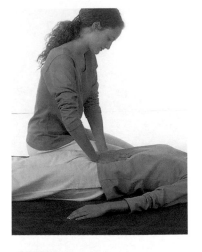

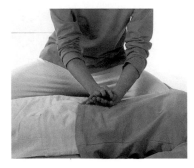

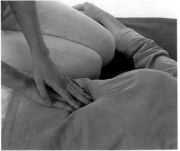

2 Using one hand on top of the other, apply pressure in a clockwise movement around the stomach. If you find tension, increase the pressure until it dissolves.

3 With one hand on the other, rock and push from one side of the belly to the other, pulling back with the heel of the hand until you feel the stomach relax.

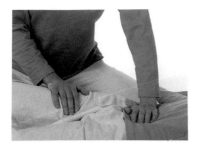

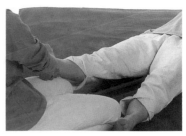

4 Stretch your partner's leg out and place your knee or a pillow underneath your partner's knee for support. Apply palm pressure along the outside frontal edge of the leg following the Stomach meridian. Start from the top of the thigh and work down to the foot.

5 Move down to your partner's feet and take a firm hold of the right ankle. Lean back and stretch the leg out. Repeat with the other leg. To finish the treatment, come back to the "hara" (abdomen) and tune in again, checking for any tension and relaxation of the muscles.

REIKI INDIGESTION TREATMENT

These hand positions aid the digestion of food and can also help to free any blockages that are caused by emotional problems – often a cause of bad digestion.

Kneel beside your partner and place one hand on the sternum and the other on the solar plexus at the centre or bottom of the rib-cage. If there is a stomach upset, constipation or diarrhoea, place the second hand lower down on the second chakra. Focus your attention and channel healing energy to the area.

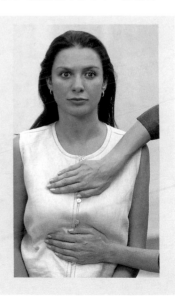

lieving stress

When we are under stress, the body pumps extra adrenalin in its "fight or flight" response. If this goes on for extended periods of time it has a damaging effect on our health and results in many common complaints.

REFLEXOLOGY EASY BREATHING

When we are stressed, our breathing becomes quick and shallow and our digestion is upset. By breathing more deeply and slowly, we can help ourselves to cope with stress: it is not possible to panic while you are breathing well. This reflexology treatment works to open up the chest and lungs. It will calm you down, settle your nerves and increase the supply of life-giving oxygen to the body.

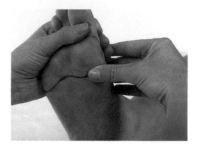

1 Thumbwalk along the diaphragm line to release tension, pain and tightness. When it is contracting and relaxing freely, the abdominal organs are also stimulated.

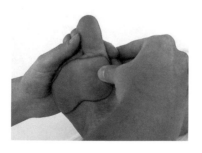

2 Work the lung reflexes on the chest area so that once the diaphragm is relaxed, the breathing can open up increasing the supply of oxygen to the body.

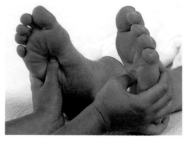

3 Take both feet together and position your thumbs in the centre of the diaphragm line. As your partner breathes in, press in with your thumbs. Release as they breathe out. Repeat this several times.

SHIATSU SHOULDER MASSAGE
Stress causes the neck and shoulders to tighten, creating pain and stiffness. This treatment gives relief.

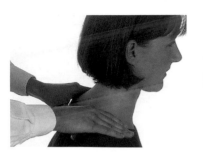

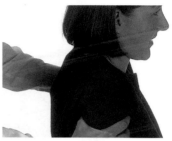

1 Place your hands on your partner's shoulders and take a moment to tune in. Grip and hold the shoulder muscles on each side of the neck. Squeeze them a few times in a rhythmic kneading action.

2 Take a firm grip of the upper arms. Ask your partner to breathe in as you lift the shoulders up and breathe out as you allow the shoulders to drop back down again. Repeat the shoulder lift three times.

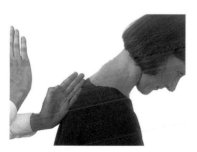

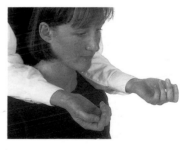

3 Use a gentle hacking action with the sides of your hands. Move rhythmically across the shoulders and base of the neck. Keep the movement consistent, then increase the intensity as you feel the muscles relax.

4 Place your forearms on your partner's shoulders. As you breathe out, press down with your arms on to the shoulders, applying gentle but firm, perpendicular, downward pressure. Repeat several times.

relieving tension

 Tension held in the body is usually the result of stress, pain or shock. The muscles tense or tighten up in an attempt to ward off the unpleasant stimuli. The healing touch of another's hands can help us to relax.

HEAD AND NECK MASSAGE

When we feel tension, we usually hold it in our shoulders and neck, keeping ourselves taut. This unnatural posture can result in a thumping headache and aching around the eye area.

A good head massage helps the facial muscles relax and worry lines disappear. You may be able to make your partner look almost 10 years younger with this tension-relieving treatment.

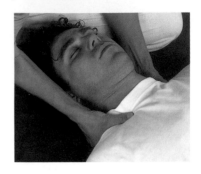

1 Place your hands on the shoulders, fingers underneath and thumbs on top. Firmly massage the shoulders using a kneading action.

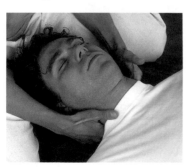

2 Move your hands to the neck. With your thumbs on the side and fingers underneath, stretch out the neck by gently pulling away. Repeat several times.

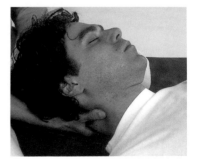

3 Lift your partner's head off the floor and firmly squeeze the muscles of the neck.

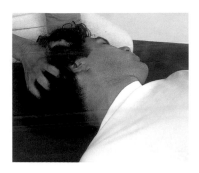

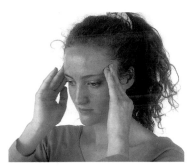

4 Rub the scalp using your fingertips and then run your fingers through the hair.

5 Using the fingers of both hands, work on the delicate facial tissue, moving symmetrically across the face to cover all the facial muscles.

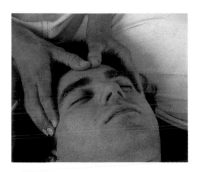

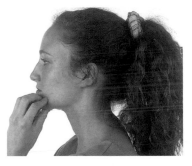

6 Place the thumbs side by side on the centre of the forehead and stroke out to the temples, working in strips. Smooth any worry lines.

7 Take the chin between thumb and fingers and gently pinch your way out along the jaw, relaxing and releasing any tension.

TIPS FOR RELIEVING TENSION

- Take regular exercise to help diffuse tension and change the focus of your attention from any worries.

- Set aside some quiet time for yourself each day.
- Unwind in an aromatherapy bath before you go to sleep.

improving sleep

A good night's sleep is essential for health. During sleep the body's cells renew and repair themselves and we relax. To prepare yourself for sleep, help the body to unwind before going to bed.

RESTFUL SLEEP ENHANCER

A foot massage and reflexology treatment will help the body to relax. It will also improve the circulation and accelerate the removal of toxins. Try this treatment to make the most of the healing properties of sleep.

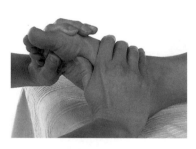

1 Holding the foot with one hand, bring the foot down on to the thumb of your other hand and lift it off again. Move your thumb one step to the side and repeat, working your thumb methodically across the foot to the outer side, following the boundary line of the ball of the foot.

▸ **3** Thumbwalk along the spinal reflex from the heel to the big toe. Support the outside of the foot with your other hand.

2 Firmly thumbwalk along the diaphragm line. It is important to relax the diaphragm, because this area helps to calm the whole body and to steady the breathing.

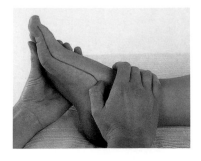

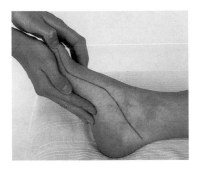

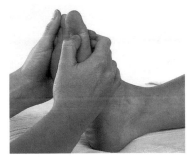

4 Repeat, going down the spinal reflex several times. Rotate gently around any tight or sensitive areas.

5 Gently thumbwalk up the back of the toes: do this with care as there is likely to be tenderness there.

AROMATIC HAND AND FOOT MASSAGE

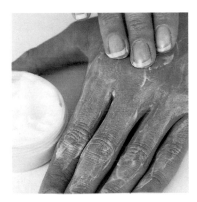

Massaging the hands and feet will help to relax the whole body. Use small, circling strokes on the soles and palms, repeating the movements on the other foot and hand. Use firm pressure to avoid tickling and irritating movements.

SLEEPY-TIME AROMAS

Try adding a few drops of essential oil to your massage oil or lotion.
• Lavender: for relaxing and balancing.
• Camomile: for soothing and calming.
• Neroli: for calming stress and anxiety.
• Clary sage or marjoram: for a strong sedative action.

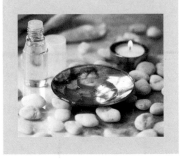

looking after your hands

We rely on our hands to perform countless everyday tasks. Our hands are one of the most overworked parts of the body, yet it is easy to take them for granted, forgetting to give them the care they deserve.

SIMPLE HANDCARE

Everyday of our lives our environment has an impact on our hands. Freezing winter temperatures, biting winds, central heating, water, detergents and strong sunlight all have a damaging effect on the delicate skin of our hands. As we get older, our skin loses its elasticity and becomes increasingly dry.

There are a few simple things that we can do to look after our hands. Exposure to the sun is believed to be the main cause of skin aging, so it's essential to protect your hands from the damaging effect of the sun's harmful

▼ USE A MOISTURIZER CONTAINING A SUN-SCREEN TO PROTECT YOUR HANDS FROM ULTRAVIOLET LIGHT AND TO KEEP THE AGING EFFECTS OF THE SUN AT BAY.

NAIL & HANDCARE TIPS

• To remove dead skin cells: add a teaspoon of salt to warm olive oil and massage into the hands.
• To strengthen the nails: rub a little neat lavender oil into the cuticles every night.
• For dry, brittle or weak nails, or nails with white flecks: make sure you have enough calcium, zinc and B vitamins.

ultraviolet rays: use a good-quality moisturizer containing ultraviolet filters. Get into the habit of wearing rubber gloves for washing up and always use a moisturizer after exposing them to water.

Age spots on the back of the hands are made worse by cold weather and sunlight. Protect your hands from wintry winds by investing in warm gloves, and use a richer moisturizer at this time of the year. Saffron oil or a few drops of lemon juice mixed into yogurt and rubbed into the hands can help to reduce age spots.

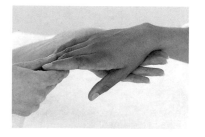

AROMATHERAPY PAMPERING TREATS
As well as looking after our hands on a day-to-day basis, a weekly manicure will keep the nails in good shape. Use essential oils to strengthen your nails.

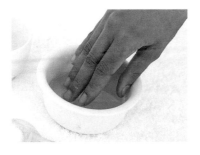

1 Soak your fingertips in either warm water, warm olive oil or use cider vinegar if the nails are weak. Gently clean the surplus cuticle from the nail area.

▼ HANDS THAT ARE NEGLECTED AND WORN-LOOKING ARE SAID TO AGE A WOMAN.

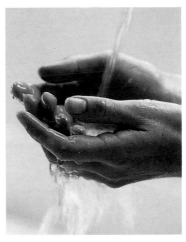

2 Gently push the cuticles back with an orange stick wrapped in cotton wool. Use a cotton bud (Q-tip) to apply neat lavender oil to each cuticle.

▼ FOR CRACKED, DRY SKIN MIX PATCHOULI OIL IN A CARRIER OIL AND APPLY TO HANDS.

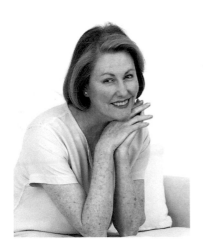

index

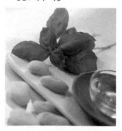